Blood Pressure Solution

Lower your Blood Pressure without Medication using Natural Remedies

By Jessica Robbins

Blood Pressure Solution

Published in the United States by Awesome Life Resources. 2015

Ebook ASIN: B00KOUV00A

Paperback: 978-1507759448

FREE AUDIO BOOK

Access the Free Audio Book version of Blood Pressure Solution by viewing the below link:

http://forms.aweber.com/form/68/20091268.htm

Format: .mp3

Size: 16.4 mb

Duration: 58 mins 44 secs

Table of Contents

Introduction

Understanding Blood Pressure

What is Blood Pressure?

Who is at Risk of Developing High BP?

Blood Pressure and Diabetes – The Connection

Blood Pressure and Coronary Heart Problems

Facts and Causes of High Blood Pressure

What causes High Blood Pressure?

Damage Caused by Blood Pressure

High BP Facts – The Silent Killer

Benefits of Lowering High BP

Natural Blood Pressure Solutions

Nature Vs Medicine

Home Blood Pressure Monitor

Revamping your Diet

Watch your Waistline

Pile on the Essential Minerals and Supplements

Exercise for an Active Lifestyle

Keep Away from Stress

Say No to Smoking and Drinking

Herbal Remedies

Switching Cooking Oils

Stress Relief Techniques

Bonus Chapter

DASH Diet Recipes

Conclusion

Thank You!

Disclaimer

Preview of "Oil Pulling Therapy: Detoxify, Heal & Transform your Body through Oil Pulling"

Introduction

Every time you visit a doctor, for an eye infection or a bad stomach, one of the first things the nurse does is - check your blood pressure. Nine out of ten times, the reason you visit the doctor is not even remotely concerned with blood pressure – high or low! Everyone who has ever visited a doctor would agree that, almost always, doctors are keen on checking their patients' blood pressure levels before proceeding with other diagnosis. You might have certainly noticed this and have, perhaps, even wondered about its necessity. However, your doctors understand the need for keeping tabs on the blood pressure of their patients.

According to the Centers for Disease Control and Prevention, one in every three American adults has high blood pressure. This is nearly 31% of the total population of the nation. While this fact is disturbing, there is yet another fact that is even more alarming – only 47% of the people diagnosed with high blood pressure have their condition completely under control. While the incidence of blood pressure varies by age, ethnicity, and sex, it, however, cannot be denied that high blood pressure costs the nation nearly $47.5 billion each year in terms of health care expenses, medications, loss of productivity and more. While it might not always be possible to convert everything into monetary loss, the sheer amount of stress and other related conditions arising from high BP can be equally daunting. It might be true that preventing high blood pressure is possible, it also quite easy to find natural and healthy solutions to tackling high blood pressure.

Understanding Blood Pressure

What is Blood Pressure?

Blood Pressure, as the name suggests, is the force of blood that is pushing against the walls of your arteries as it courses through your body. Your arteries are flexible and contractible tubes running through your body. As you know, every single time your heart beats, it pumps blood into your arteries. Just like water in a hose, your arteries can also accommodate blood only up to a certain capacity. When the pressure of blood starts increasing, your arteries won't be able to withstand the pressure; this will lead to healthy arteries being damaged and leading to life-threatening conditions such as cardiovascular diseases and stroke.

Blood pressure is highest when the heart beats and pumps out blood into the arteries. This is called systolic pressure. When the heart is between two beats, it is called as diastolic pressure. Blood Pressure reading takes these two readings and the systolic pressure reading comes before or above the diastolic pressure number. Ideally the blood pressure reading of a healthy person should be 120/80. Most medical professionals pay utmost attention to the diastolic pressure measurement because if this reading is too high, then it indicates that your heart and arteries are under too much pressure even when your heart is at rest.

If you were to take your blood pressure reading after a stint at the treadmill or after a long and tiring speech at the local school, you will notice that your blood pressure reading is nowhere near normal. This spike in blood pressure is not a cause for alarm, as it is very normal for your blood pressure to fluctuate with the changes in physical activities and emotional state of mind. Moreover, blood pressure readings also vary from person to person and even from one part of the body to another. You should be concerned when your blood pressure is consistently high; this persistent high blood pressure indicates that your heart is working far beyond its capacity. In addition to putting excessive pressure on the heart, high blood pressure also damages the arteries, kidneys, eyes and brain.

For someone to be diagnosed as having high blood pressure or hypertension, their blood pressure readings taken at least at two different occasions should be 140/90 or higher. Moreover, for those over the age of 60, even a reading of 150/90 or high might indicate high blood pressure. Those whose blood pressure readings are above 180/120 need immediate treatment.

Blood pressure is not all bad after all. The heart does exert some amount of pressure to be able to push or pump blood into the arteries so that it carries the nutrient laden blood to various parts of the body, in order to maintain healthy organs. In fact, certain amount of blood pressure is needed to provide nutrients to all parts of the body. However, too high pressure will certainly damage the arteries. With too low pressure, your heart will not be able to pump the blood to all parts of the body.

Who is at Risk of Developing High BP?

Hypertension, also known as high blood pressure, is the most common type of cardiovascular disease that is also the leading cause for stroke in people. It is also one of the major causes for heart disease. In fact, more than 30% of American adults suffer from hypertension.

There are a few common traits, habits and conditions that can raise the risk of developing high blood pressure.

Old Age: Blood pressure has a tendency to rise with age; in fact about 65% of Americans above the age of 60 have high blood pressure.

Race / Ethnicity: Although high blood pressure can affect anyone, it is, however, more prevalent among the African American population than the Caucasian or Hispanic adults.

Gender: Although men and women are equally affected by hypertension, it has been noted that before the age of 45, men are more likely to be affected by hypertension when compared to women. Moreover, after 65 years of age, women are more likely to be affected by high blood pressure.

Obesity/Overweight: People who are obese, that is have body weight that is greater than what is generally considered normal by medical professionals, have a tendency to develop high blood pressure.

Heredity: A family history of hypertension generally puts you at a risk for developing high blood pressure.

Stress and unhealthy lifestyle: Long lasting stress and an unhealthy lifestyle can also put you at a risk of developing hypertension.

Blood Pressure and Diabetes – The Connection

There is a connection between high blood pressure and diabetes as hypertension seems to be the condition that commonly affects people with Type 2 diabetes. The reason for such a connection is not very clear but it is widely assumed by medical professionals around the world that obesity, sedentary lifestyle, high sodium diet could lead to the increase in the risk of developing both the conditions.

Hypertension, commonly known as the silent killer because of a lack of easily noticeable symptoms, can be common among people already diagnosed with diabetes. Since diabetes damages the arteries by making them hard, the arteries will find it difficult to pump blood to other organs. The hardening of arteries, called atherosclerosis, hinders the free flow of blood through the arteries. If this condition is not treated, it can easily lead to kidney failure, stroke, heart attack, and heart failure.

Blood Pressure and Coronary Heart Problems

High blood pressure can develop quietly in your body for years before you start noticing its damage or symptoms. If this condition is left uncontrolled, it can lead to disability, diabetes and heart conditions. Since the heart pumps blood to all parts of the body, any form of uncontrolled pressure in the blood flow can lead to a number of fatal heart conditions. Coronary artery disease puts pressure on the arteries that supply blood to the heart muscles. As the arteries get narrowed because of coronary heart disease, blood will not be able to flow freely to and from the heart. This restricted flow causes immense pressure to build-up in the heart which can lead to chest pain and heart attack.

In addition to this, high blood pressure also forces the heart to work harder than normal to pump blood. This forces the left ventricle of the heart to stiffen or thicken, forcefully changing the ability of the left ventricle to pump blood. This condition can increase the risk of developing fatal heart conditions, heart attacks, cardiac arrests and failure. Moreover, during the course of time, prolonged strain on your heart will weaken your heart muscles. Weakened heart muscles will work less efficiently than normal and your heart will eventually wear out and stop working.

Facts and Causes of High Blood Pressure

What causes High Blood Pressure?

Although the exact causes of high blood pressure are not known, there are a few factors and conditions that contribute in the development of high blood pressure.

- Obesity or overweight
- Smoking
- Sedentary Lifestyle or Lack of Exercise
- Long Lasting Stress
- Too much Salt in Diet
- Excessive Alcohol Consumption
- Low calcium, magnesium and potassium diet
- Insulin Resistance
- Old Age
- Family history
- Chronic Kidney Disease
- Thyroid Disorders

Damage Caused by Blood Pressure

High blood pressure or hypertension is one of the main reasons for a number of health complications that can turn fatal if left untreated. Some of the complications of high blood pressure are:

- Coronary Artery Disease
- Enlarged Heart
- Arrhythmias
- Cardiac Arrest
- Heart Attack
- Heart Failure
- Atherosclerosis
- Aneurysm
- Stroke
- Dementia
- Transient Ischemic Attack
- Mild Cognitive Impairment
- Kidney Failure
- Optic Neuropathy
- Retinopathy
- Sleep Apnea
- Bone Loss

High BP Facts – The Silent Killer

The reason why high blood pressure is often called as the silent killer is because there are not many apparent symptoms of high blood pressure. In fact, most of the people diagnosed with hypertension do not know that they have high blood pressure, and by the time they are diagnosed, they would have lived with it for years without undergoing any treatment.

So, it is important to know why learning about high blood pressure is important.

- According to Centers for Disease Control and Prevention, more than 348,000 deaths reported in 2009 in America indicated high blood pressure as one of the primary contributing factors.
- This report also suggests that there were at least 1000 deaths each day because of conditions related to high blood pressure.
- In fact, seven out of every ten persons who had their first heart attack also suffered from high blood pressure.
- Nearly eight out of every ten persons who had their first stroke also have high blood pressure.
- Moreover, about seven out of every ten persons diagnosed with chronic heart failure also have high blood pressure.
- In addition to this, kidney failure is also seen to be a major risk factor for high blood pressure.

Benefits of Lowering High BP

There are a number of health benefits of lowering blood pressure. First benefit is your heart; your heart will thank you for taking care to reduce its pressure. Moreover, you get to live a healthy and active life.

According to the American Heart Association, nearly 74.5 million American adults have hypertension. As high blood pressure rarely shows signs or symptoms, this potentially dangerous condition often goes unnoticed. Therefore, it is important to lower your blood pressure to acceptable levels – 120/80. In addition to improving your overall health, maintaining your blood pressure levels at 120/80 will also help reduce your risk of developing high blood pressure related complications.

- Reducing your blood pressure levels can help you avoid heart conditions. High levels of blood pressure put an undue pressure on your heart and, increased the chances of developing peripheral artery disease, angina, coronary artery disease, heart failure and heart attack.
- Maintaining your blood pressure at healthy levels can help reduce the risk of developing a stroke. When a blood vessel to the brain becomes damaged or bursts, it causes a stroke. Chronic high blood pressure is a risk factor associated with hemorrhagic stroke and high blood pressure is a risk factor for ischemic stroke.

- Reducing the levels of blood pressure in your body helps you maintain the health of your kidneys. Your kidneys produce a hormone that is vital in maintaining the levels of blood pressure in your body. Blood pressure also damages the kidneys. Since they can no longer produce enough amounts of blood pressure regulating hormone, you can no longer regulate the levels of your blood pressure.

- Reducing the levels of blood pressure in your body helps you improve your vision. When you bring your blood pressure to acceptable levels, you reduce the strain on your optic nerves. This helps you reduce the risk of developing hypertensive retinopathy.

Natural Blood Pressure Solutions

Nature Vs Medicine

The means and methods to treat various health conditions, these days, are not confined to conventional medication alone. There are a number of health conscious people, including doctors and other medical professionals, who have claimed to have used natural treatments and remedies to counter high blood pressure – and with some really good results.

While many doctors prescribe medications when your blood pressure is consistently above 140 / 90, they generally advice you to adhere to a low-sodium diet, exercise, large quantities of fresh fruits and vegetables, stress reduction and more. So, nature and medications seem to be the solution to reducing levels of blood pressure in the body. Even if you are under medication, it is suggested that you include natural and healthy therapies to reduce your hypertension. However, regardless of whether you are presently taking medicines for your blood pressure or not, it is advised that you consult a doctor before switching over to natural and herbal medications. High blood pressure is a serious condition and it is better you do not leave its treatment to your whims and guessing games. Moreover, just because one type of herb or one type of a fruit did wonders to someone's blood pressure, it doesn't mean that you should also try it. Please consult your doctor before making changes to your diet and lifestyle.

Home Blood Pressure Monitor

High Blood Pressure should be regularly monitored so that you do not leave anything to chance. However, it is not possible to head to the doctor's every time you want to check your blood pressure levels. That is the reason why many doctors recommend you to invest in a home blood pressure monitoring system. In addition to regular monitoring in the doctor's office, it is also important that you keep track of your numbers at home. However, you should understand the home monitoring should not be used as a substitute for regular physician visits. In fact, home monitoring should be undertaken along with regular visits to your physician's place. Moreover, make sure that you do not discontinue the blood pressure medication prescribed by the doctor, even if your pressure levels appear normal on your home monitoring system. Always consult your doctor before making any changes to the prescribed medications.

There are a number of factors that can alter or affect your blood pressure levels. Make sure you avoid these factors when you take your blood pressure levels. It is also recommended that you try to take your blood pressure readings at the same time every day. Sometimes, your doctor might require you to take blood pressure readings several times a day just to see if the reading fluctuates during the day. Some of the factors that can affect your blood pressure readings are:

- Smoking
- Exercise
- Stress
- Cold Weather
- Certain Medications
- Caffeine

In fact, there are certain precautions you must undertake before checking your blood pressure levels at home.

- Always find a quiet and peaceful place to take your blood pressure readings.
- Sit in a comfortable position. Don't slouch or put too much pressure on any part of your body while taking pressure levels.
- Make sure you empty your bladder before taking the reading as a full bladder might affect your readings.
- Remove tight sleeved clothing or roll up your sleeves to expose your elbows. Make sure you do not wear very tight sleeved clothes.
- Be in rest for at least five to ten minutes before taking the reading. It gives you time to rest and relax.
- Make sure that your arm rests very comfortably on a table next to you. It should be at your heart level.
- Sit straight and rest your back comfortably against the chair. Your legs should be uncrossed.
- Your forearm should be on the table and your palm should be facing up.

In case you have purchased a digital monitor, it should be easier for you to take your readings. However, regardless of the machine you have purchased, you should read the instructions carefully before taking the readings.

- You should first locate your pulse. You can easily locate your pulse by slightly pressing your index and middle finger on the inner center of your elbow.
- In case, you are not able to locate the pulse easily, you can place the stethoscope head in your manual monitor or arm cuff on your digital monitor on the same area on your elbow.
- Once you have found the pulse, secure the cuff by passing the cuff through the metal loop and ease the cuff on to your arm and secure it. Make sure that the head of the stethoscope is secured over the artery firmly.
- The cuff should not be too tight or too loose; it should be a snug fit.
- The lower end of the cuff should be at least one inch above the bend of the elbow.
- Place the stethoscope in your ears and tilt it slightly forward so that you will be able to get better sounds.
- In case you are using a manual monitor, you have to hold the bulb in your right hand and the pressure gauge in your left.
- Completely close the airflow value present on the bulb by using the screw (turn clockwise).
- Slowly inflate the cuff by squeezing the bulb. This is when you might hear your pulse.

- Keep an eye on the gauge. Keep inflating until the reading is about 30 points more than the systolic pressure you expected.
- This is the point when you should not be able to hear your pulse on the scope.
- Very slowly release the pressure on the cuff, without taking your eyes off the gauge monitor. Make sure you turn the airflow valve very slowly in the counterclockwise direction.
- You should listen very carefully for the first pulse beat. Note down the reading as soon as you hear it. This reading is the force of blood against your artery walls – the systolic pressure.
- Continue to deflate the cuff very slowly.
- You should listen very carefully for the sound to disappear. Take down the reading as soon as you can no longer hear your pulse beat. This is your pressure of your blood between your heartbeats – the diastolic pressure.
- Deflate the cuff completely.

Home blood pressure monitoring is very important, but more important is for you to maintain a regular readings chart so that your doctor knows exactly what is happening to your heart. You will be able to provide your health care provider with an accurate image of your condition. The measurement taken at your doctor's office is just like an image frozen in a moment. It doesn't provide information about your heart's condition prior to the moment. Since high blood pressure doesn't show many symptoms, it is important to keep taking pressure readings at home. Moreover, blood pressure readings keep fluctuating throughout the day and it is next to impossible to keep heading to the doctor's every time. In addition to this, the readings are also influenced by a number of factors such as emotions, stress, medications, exercise and more.

In fact, some of you might be prone to experiencing anxiety when in the doctor's place. This anxiety and stress levels impact the blood pressure readings taken at the clinic. This is called 'white –coat hypertension.' In fact, the opposite is also said to happen to people who are very comfortable in the doctor's place and are stressed out outside the office. This is called 'reverse white-coat hypertension.' So, eventually, a number of false readings are prone to be taken. These false readings can lead to wrong diagnosis or over-diagnosis of high blood pressure. That is why home monitoring, in addition, to monitoring at the doctor's clinic is very important.

It is also important to calibrate your monitoring system every once in a while to ensure that you get correct readings. Make sure that you take your home monitoring system along with you once every six months to the doctors' so that you are able to identify any discrepancies in the readings.

Revamping your Diet

Eating a nutrition rich diet will help you reduce high blood pressure in your body. Whole grains, low fat dairy products, fruits and vegetables can help lower your blood pressure.

Whole Grains: Whole Grains should be one of the most important parts of your diet if you are looking to reduce high blood pressure. Brown rice, corn, barley, oats, whole wheat, and more such whole grains help in reducing blood pressure.

Avoid Processed Foods: It is better if you avoid processed foods such as potato chips, bacon, lunch meats, and frozen dinners as they are rich in sodium. Most American diets contain nearly 5000 milligrams of sodium when in fact 2000 milligrams per day is more than enough. Processed foods, such as crisps, pickles, soups, sausages, ham, bacon, and other preserved food items, contain high levels of sodium.

Limit Caffeine Intake: To reduce high blood pressure levels in your body, you should limit your intake of stimulants, such as caffeine, chocolate, white carbs such as pastas, sugar and sugary drinks, candy and more. The reason why caffeine is a taboo for any one diagnosed with high blood pressure is because caffeine is a nervous system stimulator. Thus, the agitated nerves will make the heart beat faster, thereby increasing blood pressure levels.

Take in Fresh Fruits and Vegetables: This goes without saying that large quantities of fresh fruits and vegetables is going to help you not only reduce blood pressure levels, but also improve your overall health as well. Some of the best foods that help you counter blood pressure levels in your body are **green leafy vegetables, berries, potatoes, beets, skimmed milk, bananas, oatmeal, flaxseed oil, olive oil, celery juice, apple cider vinegar, and cucumber.**

Increase Fiber Intake: Fiber cleanses your digestive system and helps control your blood pressure by keeping everything in balance. Fruits, vegetables, green leafy vegetables, nuts, legumes and whole grain products are rich in fiber.

Natural Remedies: There are a number of natural remedies that help in dealing with high blood pressure levels in the body. A number of researchers have pointed out that **garlic** has the ability to lower blood pressure levels in the body. You take one clove of garlic per day or pop in one garlic tablet to maintain blood pressure. Unsalted **sunflower seeds** are also great sources of magnesium which helps in battling blood pressure in the body. Make sure they are unsalted; and use them as a healthy snack. Chocolate might not be good for your heart, but one tiny square of **dark chocolate** every day does wonders to your blood pressure – and it doesn't increase your weight either.

Reduce Sodium: The American Heart Association recommends reducing your sodium intake to 2,300 mg and less than 1,500 mg per day if you are above 51. This measures to a little over half a teaspoon. Reducing sodium doesn't stop with reducing your intake of table salt. A number of processed foods, restaurant foods have high quantities of sodium. Consuming too much sodium can make your body retain fluids and, this increases blood pressure in your body.

Reduce Carbohydrates Intake: One of the main reasons for persistent increase in blood pressure levels is high blood sugar and insulin resistance. Consuming too much sugar-sweetened drinks, such as soda and tea can directly influence blood pressure. Although naturally occurring, sugar in fruits will not cause any problems, you should be wary of artificially sweetened drinks. You should consume enough carbohydrates as required by your body and health needs, but make sure they are kept at a minimum.

Watch your Waistline

One of the main factors that trigger a spike in blood pressure levels is body weight. A number of researchers have suggested that obesity is one of the primary reasons for high blood pressure levels. In fact, if you are able to reduce your body weight by a mere 10 pounds (nearly 4.5kgs), you will be able to drastically reduce your blood pressure levels. Moreover, losing weight also makes sure that the blood pressure medications that you are taking are more effective. However, make sure that you consult your doctor before trying any diet or weight reduction plans.

While watching your weight is important, you should also make sure you actually watch your waistline. You should not carry too much weight around your waist as it can put you at a greater risk for high blood pressure. For men, the waist should not be more than 40 inches or 102 cm. Women are at risk of getting high blood pressure if their waist is more than 35 inches. The reason why waistline is important is because the extra fat around your waist called visceral fat tends to surround vital organs in the abdomen. This leads to complications such as high blood pressure.

Pile on the Essential Minerals and Supplements

Vitamin B: Vitamins are very important for the well-being of the human body. When you take in the right quantities of Vitamin B 6, B 9, and B 12, you can help reduce homocystiene levels in the body which causes problems to the heart. These daily nutrients can be found in natural foods; however, you can use Vitamin supplements as well.

Omega -3: Omega -3 fatty acids should become a very important part of your diet as it has a number of health benefits to provide. In fact, tomatoes, potatoes, beans, dry fruits, fruits help in reducing heart conditions and blood pressure. Moreover, various types of fish such as salmon, herring, mackerel are all rich in Omega-3 fatty acids that help in lowering body fat called triglycerides and improving your overall health.

Potassium: Potassium is a very important mineral that helps in controlling sodium levels in your body. According to the American Heart Association, a diet rich in natural potassium can help reduce the levels of blood pressure in your body. It is recommended that you take in at least 4,700 mg of potassium daily. Potassium is present in a number of healthy foods such as white beans, spinach, salmon, white and sweet potatoes, bananas, and orange juice. Although potassium is essential for maintaining the right levels of blood pressure, you should consult your doctor about the appropriate levels of potassium required by your body as too much of potassium can be harmful too.

Vitamin C: According to a few leading medical researchers, high doses of Vitamin C is effective in controlling high blood pressure in the body. Vitamin C is known for its diuretic effect that helps in removing excess fluids from the body. This, in turn, helps blood vessels to relax. About 500 mg of Vitamin C is recommended as a daily dosage.

Vitamin D: According to researchers, the presence of the right amounts of Vitamin D in the body will help reduce high blood pressure. Vitamin D deficiency is known to contribute towards increasing blood pressure levels in the body. Vitamin D suppresses a few hormones and acts as an anti-inflammatory agent as well. So, it is important that you talk to your doctor to understand your daily requirements of Vitamin D.

Coenzyme Q10: Coenzyme Q10 is very important as it makes sure that the cells in the body function properly. Low levels of this substance have been reported among people with hypertension. Although it is not very clear whether or not the low levels of this substance produced by the human body is responsible for increasing blood pressure levels, it has been classified by the Natural Medicines Comprehensive Database as 'possibly effective; in treating high blood pressure. Moreover, CoQ10 might be available as a supplement over the counter, it is important that you consult your doctor before consuming it.

Exercise for an Active Lifestyle

Exercising is very important aspect of keeping your blood pressure within the acceptable levels. You have to walk for at least 20 to 30 minutes every day at a brisk pace. It is not necessary that you jog or run; however, any form of regular physical exercise is essential part of maintaining your blood pressure levels. If you are not able to find a good park to walk, you can always buy a treadmill and walk at home. Research has shown that regular physical activity of at least 30 minutes each day has the potential to reduce your blood pressure levels by at least 4 to 9 mm of mercury. You will be able to notice the effects of regular exercise almost within weeks. If you already have prehypertension – between 120/80 to 139/89 – regular exercise can help you avoid turning it into a fully blown blood pressure patient.

You should talk to your doctor about chalking out an exercise plan that is perfect for your body and health needs. Make exercising an integral part of your weight loss program. In addition to walking, you can also try to bring in other forms of physical activity; especially if you work style is sedentary. You can try swimming, aerobics, lifting weights, dancing, yoga and more. As long as you are able to stick to an exercise regimen, maintain it and continue to enjoy it, you will be able to experience immense health benefits from it.

Keep Away from Stress

It is inconceivable that a person, especially in this fast-paced world, can live without stress. However, it is important that you try to relax, de-stress and slow down. Although it is not possible to de-stress very easily, you should be able to find time to meditate, exercise, do yoga or at least watch a few good movies. Stress has the potential to raise your blood pressure levels instantly and if you are under constant stress, you can be sure of keeping up your blood pressure high too. You should try to figure out what is stressing you, your job, relationships, your health, and your finances; and find ways to fix the problems as well.

Learning how to combat stress is very important if you are looking for ways to reduce your blood pressure levels. Take up a disciplined hobby such as meditation or yoga. You can learn the basics of yoga or meditation from a trainer and then comfortably follow it from the comfort of your home. Moreover, if you are interested, you can also join a yoga group. Some people believe that group session helps them de-stress easily than working out on their own. In addition to helping you de-stress, yoga also has a number of asanas or postures that are believed to help reduce blood pressure levels in you.

Other than yoga, there is yet another stress-relieving technique that is very effective – deep breathing technique. All you have to do is sit in a calm and comfortable place, close your eyes and take deep breathes for about 15 minutes every day. This will work wonders to reduce your stress and in turn bring your levels of blood pressure down. Some advanced Stress Relief techniques will be discussed in the coming chapters of the book.

Say No to Smoking and Drinking

There are studies to show that smoking increases blood pressure levels in the body for up to an hour after your finish smoking. For heavy and continuous smokers, there are chances that your blood pressure levels stay elevated for longer periods of time. Moreover, heavy smokers who are already diagnosed with high blood pressure are at an increased risk for developing very high levels of blood pressure. In fact, non-smokers – second hand smokers – are also at an increased risk for developing blood pressure.

Although enjoying a glass of wine with your dinner is perfectly alright and even advised for good health benefits, it is; however, not advisable to drink alcohol in excess. Drinking more than moderate amounts can lead to a number of health conditions, most prominently, increasing blood pressure levels in the body by a number of points. Moreover, alcohol has the potential to reduce the overall effectiveness of your blood pressure medications as well.

To reduce your intake of alcohol, you can try keeping a drink diary that can help you keep track of your drinking habits. If you are planning to eliminate your drinking habit, you should try tapering off your drink over a course of two to three weeks. Instead of trying to abruptly stop your drinking, you can take help from trained professionals who will assist you to find a way to stop your habit. Moreover, binge drinking is also unhealthy; as drinking more than 3 or 4 drinks in a row can spike up your blood pressure levels immediately and also lead to a number of health problems.

Herbal Remedies

There are many ways to treat high blood pressure but, if you are interested in looking at traditional and natural ways to treat hypertension you have a number of options to choose from. If you are thinking of turning to herbal or natural home remedies as a solution or a supplement to your medication, you should first consult a doctor. You might be allergic to certain herbs; and there are a few herbs that might interfere with your medication.

<u>28 Super Foods for Hypertension</u>

Drink Hibiscus Tea: Hibiscus is a small tree that has red flowers. These flowers are rich in minerals, flavonoids and other healthy nutrients. This flower when brewed into tea has a fruity taste that works both as a cold and hot beverage. Research has shown that it reduces high blood pressure in people. Although the tea is delicious by itself, you can add honey as a sweetener.

Hawthorn Tea: Hawthorn tea is also suggested to be effective against high blood pressure. The hawthorn plant is said to have been used to treat heart conditions since the first century. This plant, rich in antioxidants, is said to be effective in opening up blood vessels in the body, thereby increasing the flow of blood through them.

Gotu Kola Tea: Gotu Kola tea is also suggested to be an effective in reducing blood pressure levels in the body. It is believed that Gotu Kola is effective in preserving the connective tissues in the body.

Moreover, it also strengths veins and improves blood circulation in the body.

Green Tea: Green tea is known for its effective blood pressure reducing properties. Being a very effective anti-oxidant, drinking a minimum of two and a half cups of green tea per day has the potential to reduce the risk of high blood pressure by at least 46 %.

Although there are varieties of tea that have the potential to reduce blood pressure levels, you can choose the right tea according to your taste and doctors' advice.

Basil: Basil is a wonderfully delicious and tangy herb that can be added to your fresh salads, soups, casseroles, pastas and more. Certain studies have shown that the extracts of basil reduce blood pressure levels in the body.

Bananas: Known for being the best on-the-go snack, Bananas are, perhaps, one of the best choices for countering high blood pressure. Bananas are loaded with potassium that is useful in helping lower blood pressure. It helps in helping kidneys function in a better way and in balancing out the effects of salt in the body. One recent study suggests that consuming two bananas everyday can help reduce your blood pressure by nearly 10%. Other foods that have high concentrates on potassium are dates, potatoes, and avocados.

It is a great functional fruit that makes a great breakfast choice or a wonderful evening treat. Better still, slice bananas into several one inch pieces and freeze them. Frozen bananas are yummy.

Broccoli: Broccoli might not be your favorite food, but it is rich in potassium, fiber, magnesium, calcium, and Vitamin C. These nutrients help in reducing blood pressure. One cup of broccoli provides nearly 200% of the amount of Vitamin C that you require every day. Although researchers aren't exactly sure how Vitamin C helps in reducing blood pressure, but it seems that Vitamin C helps in excreting lead that helps in relaxing the nervous system. It also helps in protecting nitric oxide – one molecule that helps in relaxing blood vessels and increasing the flow of blood.

Egg Whites: Another great blood pressure reducing breakfast ingredient is egg whites. Make sure you go easy on the yolk. Egg whites are great sources of protein and they contain a peptide that helps in lowering blood pressure. According to a study presented by the American Chemical Society, egg whites helped in lowering blood pressure as much as a low dose of general prescription drugs.

Dark Chocolate: We all know that dark chocolate has age-defying and mood enhancement properties. In a study conducted on older adults with pre-hypertension or hypertension revealed that consuming small amounts of dark chocolate every day for nearly 18 weeks reduced their hypertension by almost 20%.

Watermelon: Water melon is not the best summer fruit; it is also great blood pressure busting fruit. A group of researchers from Florida State University suggested that water melon contained one of the richest natural sources of L-citrulline. L-citrulline is very effective in regulating the flow of blood and blood pressure. Moreover, researchers were also of the opinion that the amino acids present in the fruit also had a positive effect in preventing pre-hypertension into becoming a full-scale hypertension.

Raisins: If you have hypertension, you should try not to ignore the little guys present in your favorite bagels, cookies, and sprinkled on desserts. Start making these chewy fruits into a healthy snack. In one study conducted on pre-hypertensive participants, it was noted that snacking on raisins three times a day for a period of 12 weeks significantly reduced the systolic and diastolic blood pressure in them.

Tomatoes: Tomatoes come packed with blood pressure reducing agent – lycopene. A recent Australian study indicated that by inducing at least 25 mg of lycopene in your daily diet, it is easier to lower LDL or bad cholesterol by nearly 10 percent.

You need not start gulping down tomatoes directly; you can try incorporating tomatoes into your diet intelligently. Remember that a cup of tomato juice contains almost 23 mg of lycopene or half a cup of spaghetti sauce has nearly 20 mg of lycopene.

Skimmed Milk: Skimmed milk or one percent milk does wonders to your heart. It provides immensely healthy calcium and vitamin D. These two key ingredients are helpful in bringing the blood pressure levels by nearly 3 to 10 percent. Moreover, they are also helpful in bringing about a 15 percent reduction in cardiovascular diseases.

Spinach: Spinach leaves are not only taste great in your salads and sandwiches, but they are also rich in fiber, magnesium, potassium and folate. These key ingredients help you maintain and control your blood pressure levels. Moreover, they are low in calories also.

Black Beans: Black beans have high fiber to protein ratio that makes them work wonders for regulating your blood sugar levels, lowering blood cholesterol levels and maintaining normal blood pressure.

Black beans are also rich in magnesium and fiber, both essential for maintaining good levels of blood pressure in the body. Moreover, black beans are also rich in folate or folic acid in synthetic form. Folate is a B complex vitamin helps in relaxing blood vessels and thereby improving blood flow. It, therefore, helps in lowering blood pressure levels in the body.

Unsalted Sunflower Seeds: Sunflower seeds are a treasure trove of magnesium which is helpful in dealing with your blood pressure levels. However, you should make sure that you do not eat salted sunflower seeds as they contain high doses of sodium, which is something you have to avoid if you want to bring your blood pressure levels down.

Soybeans: Soybeans make a wonderful and healthy snack. They are rich in magnesium and potassium. You should look out soybeans in their pod as it is one of the healthiest among all the beans. Simply boil them, and pop them right out of their shell into your mouth.

Cold-water Fish: As everyone knows, cold-water fish are best known for being the storehouse of omega-3 fats. Omega-3 fats are great for cardiovascular health, lowering blood pressure and helping reduce heart attack and stroke risk. Tuna, wild salmon, cod, trout, mackerel, halibut and sardines are rich in omega-3 fats.

Since our body needs omega-3 fats but doesn't have the ability to naturally produce them, it is important that

Dandelion: Dandelion is known to reduce blood pressure levels in the body, in addition to helping your eyes, liver and skin. Dandelion helps in releasing excess sodium from the body without the impacting potassium content. Since sodium restricts blood vessels, it increases blood pressure levels in the body. However, potassium helps in regulating the blood flow and that is the reason why dandelion helps regulate your blood pressure. Moreover, dandelion is also packed with magnesium which helps in dissolving blood clots. It also helps in stimulating the production of nitric oxide which helps in relaxing the blood vessels and aiding in better flow of blood throughout the body.

Cayenne Pepper: Cayenne pepper is considered by some to be one of the fastest foods to help lower blood pressure. By being a powerful vasodilator, cayenne pepper is extremely helpful in dilating your blood vessels and thereby improving your blood flow. Thus, cayenne pepper naturally improves the flow of blood throughout your body and helps ease the pressure off arteries.

If spicy food is your cup of tea, then you can try mixing one or two teaspoons of cayenne pepper into your tea along with honey and aloe vera. This helps reduce hypertension. If this is too spicy for your taste, simply switch to cayenne pepper supplements to get the benefits.

Turmeric: Although science has barely touched the tip of turmeric iceberg, the benefits of this super herb is just now being perceived by the scientific community. Turmeric, that contains curcumin, is known to be very effective in decreasing inflammation of the body. Inflammation is a primary cause of high cholesterol and high blood pressure. By reducing inflammation throughout the body, turmeric is effective in improving cardiovascular function of the body and in maintaining healthy blood flow.

Raw Almonds: Consuming raw almonds everyday makes a significant change in your blood pressure numbers. Being a key part of the DASH diet, raw almonds come packed with mono-unsaturated fats. These mono unsaturated fats are proven to be effective in reducing blood cholesterol levels, reducing arterial inflammation and thereby, reducing blood pressure levels in the body.

Although raw almonds have high levels of fat and calories, they help in promoting the development of lean muscles. They also promote weight loss, which means that they naturally help in promoting healthy blood circulation. When you eat raw almonds with other DASH diet prescribed nuts such as walnuts, almonds become one of most useful cardiovascular super foods.

Raw Cacao: Raw Cacao is a very effective blood pressure fighting agent as it is rich in flavonoids and a number of other anti-inflammatory agents. The flavonoids present in raw cacao act as adaptogen which help you deal with stress. Since stress is one of the common causes of hypertension, raw cacao is effective in reducing blood pressure levels in the body. Moreover, adaptogen also help in regulating the stress levels in the body which helps in regulating the blood pressure levels in the body.

There have been a number of studies conducted to study the impact of raw cacao on fighting blood pressure and it has been established that cacao flavonoids help in reducing the blood pressure levels by 4.7/2.8 mm/Hg. In addition to this, raw cacao also helps in preventing stroke and other heart diseases which normally are linked with high blood pressure.

Cinnamon: Cinnamon is a tasty and aromatic seasoning that can be added to your cereal, curries, stew, stir fries, and oatmeal. You can also try adding it to your coffee. Consuming cinnamon daily has shown considerable effect in reducing blood pressure levels.

Cardamom: Cardamom is an aromatic seasoning that has been shown to have positive effect on reducing blood pressure levels in people. You can sprinkle powdered cardamom into soups, stews, baked items and more. It not only adds a lot of aroma and flavor to the preparation, it also helps in improving your health.

Garlic: Garlic might turn you off with its pungent smell, but garlic has a lot of wonderful health benefits for those looking to reduce their blood pressure levels. Garlic is known for its ability to relax and dilate your blood vessels. Your blood vessels will start allowing more blood to flow freely to all parts of your body, thereby reducing blood pressure. Garlic can be added to a number of dishes, either raw or roasted. If you think you won't be able to eat this stuff, you can simply get yourself garlic supplements.

Celery Seeds: Celery seed is an excellent herb that has been used by the Chinese to treat hypertension. In fact, studies have proven that the consumption of celery seeds have the potential to treat hypertension. You can use the celery seeds to flavor your soups, casseroles, and stews. In addition to adding these seeds to favor your dishes, you can also make juice using the whole plant. Celery, being a diuretic, is an excellent herb that can treat hypertension.

Cat's Claw: Cat's claw, a herbal medicine, has long since been used by the Chinese to treat high blood pressure. Studies on cat's claw indicate that it may be effective in reducing high blood pressure by acting on the calcium present in your cells.

Switching Cooking Oils

Sesame Oil: Sesame oil has a number of health benefits that not only help reduce your blood pressure levels but also improve your general health. Sesame oil is rich in mono and polyunsaturated acids also called as PUFAs. These acids cut down the production of cholesterol. Moreover, sesame oil is also low in saturated fats. There are two very effective antioxidants present in sesame oil called sesamin and sesamol.

According to a recent study conducted by the American Heart Association on 195 men and 133 women with high blood pressure, it was noted that despite taking common blood pressure medication, all these people still had moderate blood pressure levels. Once this group was asked to switch to sesame oil, their blood pressure levels reduced considerably and dropped into the normal range.

The reduction in blood pressure was attributed to the presence of Vitamin E, sesamin and poly-unsaturated fatty acids in sesame oil. It was also suspected that the presence of sesamin, sesamol or both contributed to the lowering of blood pressure levels in the body.

Olive Oil: Olive oil has a lot of health benefits and its anti-hypertension properties are wonderful. On a test conducted on a number of hypertensive patients, it was noted that those who used olive oil as the only fat in their diet, were able to lower their blood pressure readings significantly. Moreover, a number of patients were also able to reduce their hypertensive drugs to a large extent.

The polyphenols available in olive oil are very effective antioxidants that protect the potentially harmful form of cholesterol such as LDL from getting oxidized. Since LDL cholesterol harms you only after it gets oxidized, olive oil helps prevent the development of atherosclerosis, cardiovascular diseases and blood pressure.

Canola: Canola, made from crushed canola seeds, is one of the healthiest cooking oils. It has one of the lowest saturated fat content and high in healthy unsaturated fats as well. It is rich in omega-3 fatty acids alpha-linolenic acid that the human body cannot produce naturally. There have been studies that suggest that the intake of canola oil daily has the potential to reduce the risk of heart conditions.

Safflower: Although studies to understand the potential of safflower oil is going on, it has been suggested that safflower oil have the properties that impact coronary heart conditions, blood pressure, Type 2 Diabetes.

The presence of vitamin E helps the body eliminate the number of free radicals, and lowering heart diseases. Moreover, safflower oil is high in unsaturated fats and low in saturated fats, both properties that make it better for your heart. In fact, omega-3fatty acids help burn excess fat, control muscle contractions, help improve immune system, and balance blood pressure levels in the body.

Soybean Oil: Soybean oil has a very distinct soy smell and it has been consistently used by the Chinese to improve their heart's health. It is rich in Vitamin D and E and polyunsaturated fatty acids. Moreover, the bean phospholipids help your brain and nerves.

Sunflower Oil: Sunflower packs in a lot of health benefits as it is packed with unsaturated fatty acids. It has the goodness of two fatty acids – the alpha-linolenic acid and the linolenic acid. The linolenic acid helps reduce cholesterol in your body and the alpha-linolenic acid has the potential to transform into DHA that can help fetal brain growth.

Stress Relief Techniques

Autogenic Training: Autogenic training has immense health benefits as it teaches your body to produce a sense of warmth and a feeling of heaviness throughout your body. It helps you experience a state of physical relaxation, body health and mental peace. Autogenic training is better than simple muscle relaxation techniques.

When you become proficient, autogenic training helps in overcoming addictions such as smoking, changing behaviors such as nail biting, mitigating physical ailments, and resolving phobias. Autogenic training helps in relieving tension, and helping you cope with environmental stimulation by removing it from your attention instead of making you feel overwhelmed by the stress. In fact, autogenic training can help bring in psychological and physiological well-being.

Autogenic training should be done every day for at least 15 minutes, in the morning, lunch, and in evening. At every session, you are required to repeat a set of visualizations that can help induce a state of relaxation. You can practice autogenic training while lying down or sitting. It is important to practice autogenic training in a quiet place, and while wearing loose clothing. Initially, you might be required to lie down while performing this technique but you can change your posture after you understand the technique. Moreover, you should also avoid drinking, eating or smoking during practicing.

Always start the training with a warm up and make sure you actually feel the benefits of each stage. Be prepared to repeat the same stage if you don't completely feel relaxed after completing the stage. Since autogenic training brings in a number of benefits to you – especially helping you relax – it is very useful in alleviating your blood pressure levels.

Biofeedback: Biofeedback, as the name suggests, uses your mind to keep your body functions in control. Biofeedback helps you get connected to electrical sensors that help you receive messages from your body. With the feedback from your body, you would be able to better understand the subtle changes happening in your body and also focus on making changes to your body such as relaxing a few muscles, reducing pain and achieving the results that you want.

Biofeedback gives your mind and thoughts to deal with controlling, and healing your physical and mental condition. It is seen as a relaxation technique, it is non-invasive, reduces the need for medication, and is seen by many as an alternative treatment.

Biofeedback session begins when the therapist attaches a number of electrical sensors to various parts of your body. These electrical sensors keep track of your physiological state of your body such as temperature, brain waves, muscular tension and more. This information is given to you in the form of sound or light cues. You will be required to change your thoughts, behavior or emotions. If you are suffering from incessant headaches, biofeedback can help you focus on relieving the tension present in those particular muscles that relate to your headaches.

Biofeedback session lasts anywhere between 30 to 60 minutes. The duration of the session depends largely on the conditions you want to heal and the control you want to gain.

Qi Gong: Qi Gong, sometimes also called as Chi Kung, is a health regimen that consists of simple, plain and easy movements. Plain breathing exercises that can be performed while you are lying down or sitting comfortably helps in reliving body tension and pressure. Breathing as if you are planning to blow out a candle or breathing in a way that you mimic the hiss of a snake, Qi Gong practitioners believe that you are able to take in energy through your body's natural pathways called the meridians.

Qi Gong makes use of breath, mind, and simple movements to develop a clear, calm and balanced energy that can be used to relax, rejuvenate and heal. There are two types of Qi Gong – the soft and the hard Qi Kong. Tai Chi is a form of the soft Qi Gong also called as the inner Qi Gong.

Qi Gong involves using moving meditation, slow rhythmic movements, deep breathing, and meditative mind. Qi Gong's techniques are based on intentional movements where you move your body in a careful and free flowing manner, rhythmic breathing where you breathe in a slow and controlled manner, visualization of the flow of qi or chi, awareness of the mind's meditative state, and chanting. Since Qi Gong combines and streamlines the body, mind and breath, it is considered to be very useful in improving respiratory and cardiovascular functions of the body.

"T'ai Chi: Unlike the common perception of martial arts where there is constant punching, kicking and fighting, "t'ai chi is a slow, rhythmic and controlled body movement technique that helps you gain inner peace and calm.

There are two features of "t'ai chi training, one is the 'solo' form and the other is 'pushing hands' form. The solo form is a sequence of slow movements which emphasize the need for a straight spine and natural movements. The other pushing hands form involves training with a partner, sensing their movements and producing appropriate responses using your hands.

"T'ai chi helps ease your inner muscles, controls the central nervous system, releases stress – both physical and mental – and promotes a feeling of spiritual, physical and mental well-being. It tones down the muscles, releases built-up tension, and relaxes the knots and stress in them. It is known to be effective in helping you deal with chronic heart conditions, diabetes, depression, and blood pressure.

Bonus Chapter

DASH Diet Recipes

Before we look to DASH diet recipes, we need to know a little about DASH diet and its effectiveness in controlling and reducing high blood pressure. DASH – Dietary Approaches to Stopping Hypertension – is a diet that has been proved to be effective in reducing blood pressure, and improving the overall health and lifestyle of people. In fact, DASH diet is not only effective in reducing hypertension, it works on reducing total cholesterol and low-density lipoprotein as well. Here is a sample DASH diet that includes breakfast, lunch and dinner recipes:

Breakfast:

Soup:

Gingery Chicken Noodle Soup

This soup, per serving, has 11 g total carbohydrates, 267 mg sodium, 5 g total fat, and 184 calories.

Ingredients Required:

Dried Soba Noodles – 3 ounces

Chopped Yellow Onion – 1

Peeled and finely chopped carrot – 1

Peeled and minced fresh ginger - 1

Minced garlic – 1 clove

Chopped skinless and boneless chicken breast – 1 pound

Chicken stock or broth – 4 cups

Shelled edamame – 1 cup

Sodium reduced soy sauce – 2 tablespoons

Plain soy milk – 1 cup

Olive Oil – 1 tablespoon

Chopped fresh cilantro – ¼ cup

Preparation:

- Boil ¾th cup water in a saucepan.
- Add noodles and cook till tender.
- Drain and set aside.
- Heat olive oil over medium heat in a large saucepan.
- Add chopped onion, ginger, carrot and sauté.
- Add garlic and sauté.
- Add the chicken stock, soy sauce and bring to boil.
- Add chicken and edamame and bring to boil.
- Reduce heat and simmer until chicken and edamame is tender.
- Add the remaining noodles, soy milk and cook. Don't boil.
- Remove from heat and stir in chopped cilantro.
- Serve hot.

Sandwich:

Portobello Mushroom Burger

One Portobello mushroom burger has 45 g total carbohydrate content, 9 g total fat, 163 mg sodium, and 301 calories in total.

Ingredient Required:

Portobello mushroom caps – 4 large

Minced garlic – 1 clove

Water – ½ cup

Balsamic Vinegar – 1/3 cup

Cayenne Pepper – ¼ teaspoon

Toasted whole wheat buns – 4

Tomato – 4 slices

Red Onion – 4 slices

Bibb lettuce leaves – 2 halved

Sugar – 1 tablespoon

Olive oil – 2 tablespoons

Preparation:

- Clean the mushrooms thoroughly with a dampened cloth and remove their stems.
- Place these in a glass bowl with their gill side up.

- In a small bowl, whisk vinegar, water, pepper, sugar, garlic, olive oil together.
- Pour this marinade over the mushrooms.
- Cover the bowl, marinate in the refrigerator for about an hour.
- Heat a gas grill or a broiler (or you can also use a charcoal grill)
- Lightly coat the grill rack with cooking spray.
- Place the rack at least 4 to 6 inches from the heat source
- Grill the mushrooms on a medium flame for about 5 minutes each side until they are cooked.
- Make sure to baste the marinade to keep them moist while cooking.
- Transfer the mushrooms to a plate using tongs
- Neatly place one tomato slice, one onion slice, one half lettuce leaf on top of each mushroom on a bun and serve.

Lunch:

Roasted Salmon with Maple Glaze

One fillet of roasted salmon with maple glaze has about 14 g of total fat, 152 mg of sodium, 25 g protein, and 314 calories.

Ingredients Required

Salmon– 2 pounds

Fresh cracked black pepper – 1/8th teaspoon

Minced garlic – 1 clove

Maple syrup – ¼ cup

Kosher or sea salt – 1/4 tablespoon

Fresh mint – As required

Preparation:

- Preheat oven to 450 F.
- Coat the baking pan with cooking spray.
- Mix together maple syrup, balsamic vinegar, garlic in a small saucepan over low heat. Heat until hot and remove.
- Pour half this mixture into a bowl for basting. Keep the rest aside.
- Cut salmon into 6 equal sized fillets, pat salmon dry, keep skin side down on the baking sheet, smoothly brush it with maple syrup mixture.
- Bake for about 10 minutes. Remove it. Brush with maple syrup mixture. Bake for another 5 minutes.
- Bake and baste until fish starts to flake easily – 20 to 25 minutes in total.
- Place these salmon fillets on plates. Sprinkle salt and pepper and pour the reserved maple syrup over this.
- Garnish with mint.
- Serve immediately.

Dinner:

Baked Chicken with wild rice, onion and tarragon

One serving (about 2 cups) of baked chicken with wild rice, onion and tarragon contains nearly 37 g total carbohydrates, 3 g total fat, 180 mg sodium, and 330 calories.

Ingredients Required:

Boneless, skinless chicken breast halves – 1 pound

Whole pearl onions – 1 ½ cups

Chopped celery – 1 ½ cups

Uncooked long grain rice – ¾ cup

Uncooked wild rice – ¾ cup

Unsalted chicken broth – 2 cups

Fresh Tarragon – 1 teaspoon

Dry White wine – 1 ½ cups

Preparation:

- Preheat oven to 300 F
- Chop the chicken breasts into 1 inch pieces
- Take a nonstick frying pan – add chicken, pearl onions, celery, and tarragon along with one cup unsalted chicken broth.
- For about 10 minutes, cook on medium heat until the vegetables and chicken are tender.
- Set this aside to cool.
- Soak wine, rice and remaining chicken broth for about 30 minutes in a baking dish.
- To this baking dish, add the cooked and cooled chicken and vegetables.

- Add more broth if the rice is too dry. Keep checking periodically.
- Serve immediately.

Salad:

Salad greens with fennels, pears and walnuts

One serving of salad greens with fennels, pears and walnuts contains 10 g of total fat, 3 g protein, 14 g total carbohydrates, and 50 mg of sodium.

Ingredients Required:

Mixed salad greens – 6 cups

Trimmed and thinly sliced Fennel bulb – 1 Medium

Grated parmesan cheese – 2 tablespoons

Cored, quartered and thinly sliced pears – 2 medium sized

Toasted and coarsely chopped Walnuts – ¼ cup

Balsamic vinegar – 2 tablespoons

Extra-virgin olive oil – 3 tablespoons

Freshly ground black pepper – To taste

Preparation:

- Place the salad greens into six different bowls.
- Scatter the pears and fennel all over the greens.

- Sprinkle walnuts and parmesan cheese over this mixture.
- Drizzle vinegar and olive oil.
- Sprinkle black pepper to pep up the taste.
- Serve immediately.

Conclusion

High blood pressure is one of the most commonly prevalent conditions among American adults. According to the U.S. Centers for Disease Control and Prevention, more than 67 million Americans have elevated levels of blood pressure. Blood pressure or hypertension keeps the blood pressure at constantly elevated levels, thereby changing the very structure and functions of the blood vessels. Hypertension can wreak havoc to most of our vital organs – from causing blindness to stroke. In fact, one of the main reasons for the extent of damage caused by high blood pressure is that this condition is present predominantly without clear or distinct symptoms. So, most people suffering from elevated levels of blood pressure are unaware of the condition they are suffering from. It is, no doubt, called the silent killer as it silently kills people. However, hypertension is seen primarily as a result of a bad lifestyle choice; that is the reason why most doctors lay stress on changing our habits to bring the high blood pressure numbers down.

Healthy and nutritious diet, especially DASH diet, weight reduction, avoiding sedentary work life, regular exercise, completely giving up smoking, avoiding too much alcohol, and de-stressing are sure-shot ways to reduce elevated blood pressure in your body. Moreover, there are a number of herbal and home remedies that are equally effective in dealing with hypertension. High blood pressure might not be an easy condition to get rid of;

however, with good food, active lifestyle, good health choices and mind-calming exercise, you can certainly keep the high numbers at bay.

Thank You!

Thank you for purchasing and downloading this book! I hope the book was able to help you understand the different ways to control and lower your blood pressure and motivate you enough adopt natural remedies to manage hypertension!

Finally, if you enjoyed this book, please take the time to share your thoughts and post a review on Amazon. It'd be greatly appreciated!

This feedback will help me to continue writing the kind of books that would give you the maximum value and results. Thank you once again and good luck!

FREE AUDIO BOOK

Don't forget to get access to the Free Audio Book version of Blood Pressure Solution by viewing the below link:

http://forms.aweber.com/form/68/20091268.htm

Format: .mp3

Size: 16.4 mb

Duration: 58 mins 44 secs

Disclaimer

This Book, Blood Pressure Solution: Lower your Blood Pressure without Medication using Natural Remedies is written with an intention to serve as a purely informational and educational resource. It is not intended to be a medical advice or a medical guide. Although proper care has been taken to ensure the validity and reliability of the information provided in this Book, readers are advised to exert caution before using any of the information, suggestions, and methods described in this book.

The writer does not advocate the use of any of the suggestions, diets, and health programs mentioned in this book. This book is not intended to take the place of a medical professional, a doctor and physician. The information in this book should not be used without the explicit advice from medically trained professionals especially in cases where urgent diagnosis and medical treatment is required.

Eat Well, Stay Healthy!

Preview of "Oil Pulling Therapy: Detoxify, Heal & Transform your Body through Oil Pulling"

What is Oil Pulling?

Oil Pulling is an ancient remedy for oral health problems. A traditional Ayurvedic remedy, Oil Pulling is known to work effectively in treating common oral health problems using simple and easy to use methods. Oil Pulling or Oil Swishing, as it is otherwise called, is a process of swishing oil in the mouth in order to cleanse the mouth of germs and bacteria. In addition to cleaning the mouth of germs, Oil Pulling is also known to bring in a lot more benefits to you.

According to ancient Indian health care system, Ayurveda, Oil Pulling pulls out the hidden toxins in the body and cleanses the mouth easily. When the mouth is clean, it is understood that the whole body will start reflecting it. Since our digestion starts at the mouth, when the mouth is clean and free of harmful bacteria and other germs, we can be sure that our whole body will be less likely to be affected by germs and bacteria.

Although dentistry was not treated as a specialized part in Ayurveda, it is, however, included in the section that deals with surgery. A number of tooth problems, such as oral deformities, bad breath, cavities and other infections were treated and managed in ancient India using the teachings and texts of Ayurveda. Traditional medicine has been known to treat a number of ailments and problems, without bringing on the usual side effects.

Ayurveda, a holistic system of medicine that evolved some 3000-5000 years ago in India, is now being practiced all over the world as it is an effective treatment to many common ailments. One of the main reasons for the popularity of this form of treatment, is that is easy to use, it is affordable and it does not bring in any side effects. Literature about the effects of Oil Pulling can be seen in the ancient Vedic Texts.

The concepts and ideas behind Oil Pulling are steeped in the teachings and texts of Ayurveda, where the dental health of a person is seen more as a sum total of the individual's health. It is not curtailed to the health of the mouth alone; it is seen to be very individualistic in nature. The dental health was not seen as something generic, in fact, it was seen to differ from one person to another. The individual's constitution, the climatic conditions and changes, planetary influences and more were also considered.